Fear to Freedom

I0082794

Unleashing the Power Within and Overcoming Life's Biggest Obstacles to Conquer Fear and Live Authentically: Mastering Your Inner Demons

Michele L. Valdez

Introducing the exclusive and captivating world of Michele L. Valdez. Immerse yourself in the timeless elegance and creativity that defines our brand. Experience the unparalleled craftsmanship and attention to detail that sets us apart. Discover the essence of sophistication and style with our exquisite collection. Copyright © 2024 Michele L. Valdez

Table of Contents

Preface

Greetings, Fearless Seeker

Are you sick and weary of having to live under constant fear? Do you have aspirations of realizing your full potential and escaping the chains that are keeping you back? If so, I cordially encourage you to embark on a life-changing adventure marked by bravery, resiliency, and relentless progress.

Presenting " Fear to Freedom: Unleashing the Power Within and Overcoming Life's Biggest Obstacles to Conquer Fear and Live Authentically: Mastering Your Inner Demons." This book isn't your typical self-help read. It's a sign of optimism, a path to freedom, and evidence of the limitless power within of you.

Unleash Your Inner Bully

Through the pages of " Fear to Freedom," you will set out on a journey to discover the latent strength that resides within you. You'll discover how to use the strength of your fears to turn them from roadblocks to chances for personal development. With engaging stories, useful activities, and ageless knowledge, you'll set off on a unique self-discovery adventure.

Rethink How You Interact with Fear

The days of shrinking in the face of fear are long gone. " Fear to Freedom" pushes you to rethink how you interact with fear and to view it as a tool for progress rather than an enemy. As you bravely venture into the unknown, you'll discover how to accept discomfort, face ambiguity, and dance with vulnerability.

Action-Based Empowerment

However, " Fear to Freedom" emphasizes action above simply theory. You'll learn useful methods and tried-and-true approaches for facing your anxieties and taking back control of your life. Each chapter is brimming with resources to support you on your journey, from mindfulness exercises to doable strategies for confronting your biggest fears.

Become a Part of the FearLESS Community

On your path to " Fear to Freedom," you're not going it alone. You join a thriving group of people known as warriors—those who are dedicated to live life on their own terms and who will not allow their anxieties to define them. Make connections with other seekers, discuss your victories and setbacks, and take courage from the group mentality of your fellow fighters.

Are You Prepared to Live Without Fear?

Now is the moment to break free from the bonds of fear and see your actual potential. Now is the moment to embrace your inner warrior and live the life that was planned for you. Are you prepared to go out on this once-in-a-lifetime adventure?

Bid farewell to uncertainty and welcome to possibilities. Bid farewell to inaction and hello to initiative. Bid farewell to your former self and welcome the brave warrior that resides within.

Come along on the " Fear to Freedom" trip with us and learn about your own infinite power. Is your mind set to grasp your destiny?

With bravery and steadfastness,

Introduction

Discover the untapped potential that lies within you and embark on an extraordinary transformation from Fear to Freedom with the revolutionary guide penned by the highly acclaimed author, Michele L. Valdez. Step into a world where uncertainty, anxiety, and self-doubt no longer hold you captive. Discover the transformative power of this book as it illuminates a path of hope, providing you with practical strategies to liberate yourself from the suffocating grip of fear. It's time to reclaim your life and embrace a future filled with limitless possibilities.

Introducing Fear to Freedom: The Ultimate Guide to Unlocking Your True Potential. Say goodbye to ordinary self-help books and embark on a life-changing journey towards liberation. Unlock the secrets to a life of boundless joy and fulfillment with Michele L. Valdez's groundbreaking approach. By harnessing the power of cutting-edge research in psychology, neuroscience, and personal development, Valdez offers practical insights and easy-to-follow techniques to conquer your deepest fears. Say goodbye to limitations and hello to a life of unbridled happiness.

Uncover the secrets to quieting your inner critic, conquering paralyzing anxiety, and embracing uncertainty with unwavering courage and resilience. Prepare to be moved and inspired as you embark on a transformative journey with Michele L. Valdez. In her captivating book, she fearlessly opens up about her personal struggles and triumphs, inviting readers to join her in breaking free from the shackles of fear. With each poignant anecdote and profound piece of wisdom, Valdez empowers and encourages readers to rewrite their own stories, unlocking their limitless potential. Get ready to embrace a life of boundless freedom and discover the incredible power that lies within you.

Introducing Fear to Freedom - the ultimate solution for conquering your deepest fears. No longer will you be held back by the paralyzing grip of failure, rejection, or the unknown. With Fear to Freedom, you'll be armed with powerful tools to confront your demons head-on and emerge victorious, stronger than you ever thought possible. Say goodbye to fear and hello to a life of limitless potential. Get Fear to Freedom today and unlock the path to your true greatness. Experience the liberation from sleepless nights and the shackles of self-doubt. Now is the moment to seize control and welcome the boundless opportunities that lie beyond the realm of fear.

Experience the transformative power of embracing the journey from Fear to Freedom. Today is the day to embark on a life-changing odyssey of self-discovery, empowerment, and unparalleled growth. Don't miss out on this incredible opportunity. Escape the clutches of fear and seize control of your destiny. It's time to embark on a journey towards a future filled with boundless possibilities. Experience the transformative power of Fear to Freedom and unlock the key to your success. Don't wait any longer, get your copy now and embrace the life you've always dreamed of.

Experience the exhilaration of conquering your fears and unlocking your true potential. Discover the power of personal development and self-help as you embark on a transformative journey towards resilience and empowerment. Let go of anxiety and embrace a life filled with courage, fulfillment, and self-discovery. Tap into your inner strength and cultivate psychological resilience like never before. It's time to break free from the shackles of fear and embrace a life of limitless possibilities. Introducing the brilliant mind behind the words.

C h a p t e r 1

Discover the Intriguing World of The Mindset of Fear

Discover the power of Fear, one of the most common and instinctive human emotions. Have you ever found yourself in a situation where you have to speak in front of a crowd, and suddenly you feel the pressure building up, making you fear that you might freeze or stumble? Introducing a novel approach: perhaps you yearn to express your emotions, yet find yourself consumed by the overwhelming surge of heart palpitations? Experience the powerful presence of fear, an emotion that permeates every aspect of our existence. Unlock the power of the mind and discover the hidden forces that give rise to Fear. Discover the captivating world of fear as we delve deep into its intricate workings and uncover its hidden truths.

Experience the power of fear, a captivating blend of biochemical and emotional reactions.

Discover the primal emotion that lies within every human,

a powerful tool that unveils the hidden risks lurking in our midst. Discover the ancient secret that kept our ancestors alive. Experience the fascinating world of reactions with not just one, but two distinct types: a captivating biochemical response and an intriguing psychological reaction.

Experience the power of biochemical sensations coursing through your body. Feel your heart rate quicken, the gentle sheen of sweat forming on your skin, and the surge of adrenaline heightening your senses. Embrace the physical manifestations of biochemical reactions, as they awaken your body and invigorate your being. Introducing the fascinating world of the combat or trip response! Brace yourself as your body gears up for an epic showdown or a daring escape. It's a thrilling spectacle unfolding right before your eyes. Introducing the indispensable auto-response that paves the way to triumph! Even in the most benign circumstances, we've all experienced it - that moment when beads of perspiration start to form as you gear up to deliver a monumental presentation.

Introducing the extraordinary emotional response - a tailor-made reaction to fear like no other. Embrace the thrill-seekers who fearlessly confront challenges head-on. These daring souls are what we affectionately refer to as adrenaline junkies. Discover a world where some choose to avoid any situation, while others embrace the power of fear, seeing it as both a force for good and a potential obstacle. Explore the intriguing dynamics of fear and its impact on our lives.

Unlocking the Secrets of the Mind: Unveiling the Causes of Fear

Discover the compelling rationale behind this intriguing concept. Discover the intriguing mystery behind why people are filled with fear when it comes to insects and the mysterious sounds that echo in the darkness of the night. Discover the intriguing reason behind why the mere thought of delivering an organizational presentation sends waves of nervousness coursing through your veins. Introducing a remarkable phenomenon that eludes comprehension, defies control, and instills fear of potential harm.

Introducing our exclusive range of worries, carefully crafted to cater to your every need. Discover the two exceptional types that will leave you feeling confident and in control:

Experience the thrill of natural fears.

Introducing: Conditioned Fears

Discover the extraordinary power of natural talents that are inherent from birth. Introducing the ultimate test of courage: a face-off with a majestic, powerful lion. With its immense strength and undeniable appetite, it's only natural to feel a surge of fear in such a momentous encounter. Introducing the remarkable concept of conditioned concerns - a phenomenon that occurs when a negative event from the past instills a deep fear within us, causing us to dread its recurrence. Discover the fascinating reasons behind this intriguing phenomenon. Discover the fascinating world of human psychology, where our intricate brains can sometimes play tricks on us. It's remarkable how our minds can lead us to believe that similar situations will always yield identical outcomes, even when it defies logic.

Imagine a moment from your childhood when you were innocently bitten by a playful dog. Imagine a scenario where the most joyful and adorable dog approaches you with nothing but pure friendliness in its heart. Despite its innocent intentions, it's only natural for you to have a reaction. Discover the power of making informed choices. Don't let one bad experience define your future. Embrace the possibilities that lie ahead and open yourself up to new opportunities.

Discover the power of breaking free from conditioned fear and embracing the positive. Discover the unfortunate reality of prejudice that plagues our society, causing division among people. It is a phenomenon that often arises within ourselves, perpetuating this harmful cycle. Discover the power of overcoming the influence of others. While it's true that we may not be easily swayed by the actions of those around us, there are instances where we find ourselves placing our trust in someone or perceiving something as a potential threat. In these situations, fear can creep in, even if we've never had a personal encounter with the individuals in question.

Experience the transformative power of acclimation with Reversal through Acclimation.

Discover the incredible power of conquering your fears by simply facing them head-on. Imagine the freedom and empowerment that comes from turning your fears upside down. It's time to take control and transform your life. Discover the powerful truth behind the age-old wisdom of confronting your fears head-on. While it may seem trivial at first, the reality is that facing your anxieties is the key to overcoming them.

Discover the power of confronting your deepest fears. Discover the thrilling world of insects, the mysterious allure of snakes, or the art of captivating conversations over the telephone. Imagine finding yourself in a challenging situation where you are faced with a common concern: starting a new job that requires frequent telephone communication. Experience a sense of trepidation at first, but as the days go by, you'll come to realize that the issue is actually quite relatable. Experience a remarkable decrease in the Fear response and a surge of elation with our revolutionary approach. Discover the key to overcoming concerns and treating phobias like never before. Discover the exhilarating reason why countless adrenaline junkies are irresistibly drawn to these daring escapades. Experience breeds a craving for more. Once they've tasted the thrill of risk, they yearn for bigger and bolder actions to keep their adrenaline pumping.

Discover the fascinating world of Phobias!

Experience the power of phobias, those deeply ingrained anxieties that we've all felt at some point. Experience the power of stress management and conquer your fears with ease. Experience a sense of fear? Don't let panic disorders hold you back. It's common to perceive fear as a negative response, but there's a better way. Embrace the opportunity to overcome your fears and unlock your true potential. Experience the intriguing phenomenon of phobia, a captivating twist on our natural reactions.

Delve into a world where fear takes center stage, directed towards objects or situations that may not pose any real danger. Brace yourself for a thrilling exploration of the human psyche. Introducing a remarkable solution for those struggling with this issue. While some may dismiss their concerns as irrational, they find themselves unable to overcome them. As days turn into weeks, the fear only intensifies, as the grip of anxiety tightens its hold.

Discover the fascinating world of societal concerns and levels that captivate people's attention. Dive into the intricate fabric of our society and explore the depths of its complexities. Standards, in general, are anything but ordinary and certainly not scary. Experience the ultimate peace of mind in a meticulously secured environment. With an abundance of safety measures in place, it would seem rather trivial to respond in such a way. Discover the incredible power of phobias - a force that can send shivers down your spine and intensify your fears instead of fading away.

Conquer Your Phobias and Fears with Our Expert Treatment

Unlock the power of effective management by embracing the mindset of Fear. Discover the two game-changing techniques that will revolutionize your approach:

Introducing two powerful techniques to help you overcome your fears and anxieties:

- Systemic Desensitization - A proven method that gradually exposes you to your fears in a controlled and safe environment, allowing you to build resilience and reduce your emotional response.

- Flooding - Dive

Experience the power of both to decrease your response and conquer your fears.

Experience the transformative power of systemic desensitization as it guides individuals with phobias through a series of carefully curated scenarios and exposure opportunities. Imagine a scenario where an individual is troubled by the quality of their drinking water. Introducing the captivating first program that delves into the world of drinking water. Prepare to embark on a mesmerizing journey as we explore the wonders of this life-giving elixir. Immerse yourself in the enchanting visuals of pristine drinking water, perhaps even venturing to a serene oasis. Brace yourself for an awe-inspiring finale as we conquer not one, but two majestic bodies of water. Get ready to quench your thirst for adventure! Discover the cutting-edge nature of this highly progressive process, where the key element lies in acquiring and implementing the precise strategies to effectively manage and overcome your fearful reactions. Discover effective strategies to effectively manage and overcome worries related to the problem at hand. Learn how to eliminate worrisome responses that may arise as a result of these concerns.

Introducing the undeniable phenomenon of flooding. Prepare to be amazed! This incredible opportunity has the potential to not only achieve success, but also exceed your wildest expectations. Brace yourself for a truly astonishing experience! Introducing a groundbreaking solution that empowers individuals to conquer their fears with ease. Our revolutionary approach provides a massive amount of exposure to the dreaded situation or object, allowing individuals to effortlessly acclimate to it. Say goodbye to fear and embrace a life of confidence and freedom!

Discover the power of overcoming worries and transforming your life. While worries may seem overwhelming, they don't have to define your reality. Take control of your thoughts and embrace a positive mindset that propels you towards success. Experience the transformative power that will ignite your desire to break free and seize life's opportunities. Discover how it can shape your responses to challenges and reshape your perspective on the world. Imagine a world where fear no longer holds you back. Instead of turning every risk-taking action into something terrible, you approach them with confidence and excitement. No longer confined to a defensive mindset, you are free to evaluate every opinion and make smarter decisions. Say goodbye to the limitations of fear and embrace a life of boldness and wisdom. Discover the reason why individuals experience a surge of fear and unease, caught off guard when faced with the need to make a rational decision.

Introducing an undeniable truth: when faced with fear, the mind has a tendency to perceive every situation as unfavorable. It's a natural response that cannot be ignored. Introducing the heart-wrenching reality of parenthood: imagine having a precious child who battles an unfortunate illness or endures unimaginable damage. In such trying times, the mere thought of stepping foot into a hospital can evoke a sense of fear and anxiety, among other valid concerns. Discover a world where every action is intertwined with its surroundings, creating a web of intrigue and endless possibilities. As you delve deeper, you'll find yourself making connections you never thought possible. Embrace the thrill of unraveling the mysteries that lie within. Discover the key to a healthier lifestyle and unlock the power within you. It's crucial to understand the profound impact that fear can have on both your well-being and the trajectory of your life.

Embrace Courage and Overcome Your Fears!

Introducing the undeniable truth: fear is an innate part of the human experience. However, if you find yourself drowning in a sea of excessive fear, anxiety, and stress, fret not! There are numerous strategies at your disposal to conquer these formidable foes. Discover the transformative power of seeking guidance from a skilled counselor or esteemed mental health professional to address the anxiety that burdens you. Discover the power of foresight and unlock a brighter future. Embrace the potential for change and watch as your circumstances transform into something truly extraordinary. Don't let fear hold you back - take control and create the life you've always dreamed of. Discover the power of overcoming fear with ease. While it may seem challenging at times, our expert guidance is here to provide the support you need to conquer your concerns. Embrace the opportunity to transform your mindset and unlock a world of endless possibilities.

Unlocking the Power of Overcoming Failure

Introducing a powerful mindset shift: instead of dwelling on my past failures, I have chosen to embrace them as valuable learning opportunities. By adopting the mantra "there is absolutely no failure, only opinions," I have unlocked a world of growth and resilience. I am now firmly convinced that every setback brings with it a wealth of knowledge. In fact, the lessons learned from failure are far more valuable than those derived from success alone.

Introducing the all-too-familiar struggle with failure and rejection that many of us face. Unlock your true potential and never be held back again. Don't let fear of failure stop you from reaching new heights. Embrace the possibilities and watch yourself soar. Discover the power to conquer this particular Fear by delving into its depths and charting a course to overcome its detrimental impact. Embark on a journey that promises to challenge you at every turn. Brace yourself for the obstacles that lie ahead, for they will only serve to strengthen your resolve. With unwavering determination, you will unlock the doors of your mind, inching closer to the liberating embrace of true freedom.

Discover the Origins of Your Fear of Failing

Are you one of the lucky few who grew up with overly protective parents, shielding you from the exhilarating experience of trying something new? Immerse yourself in the notion that their actions were driven by a genuine desire to do what's best for you. However, if you were to observe the situation from an objective standpoint, you would realize that it had no correlation to you whatsoever. Instead, it was all about them. Discover the transformative power of perception. By recognizing the impact of past experiences on your present, you can unlock a brighter future. Don't let the weight of stress define you any longer. Embrace the opportunity to take control and thrive in even the most challenging situations. Your life is waiting for you to seize it.

Unravel intricate problems with ease

Experience the thrill of stepping outside your comfort

zone and embracing the allure of sophistication. Discover a world of possibilities as you delve into a captivating challenge that will pique your interest. Don't let the fear of failure hold you back - instead, let it fuel your determination to conquer the seemingly impossible. Unleash your inner adventurer and embark on a journey of self-discovery. Take the first steps towards success by breaking it down into manageable items. Discover the power of learning from experience and seamlessly transitioning to the next step when faced with a setback. Embrace the wisdom gained from each part that fails, propelling you towards success. By embracing this approach, you will discover the true power of turning setbacks into opportunities for growth.

Embrace the power of failure to unlock your growth potential

Embrace the reality that failure is an inevitable part of life, regardless of your status or achievements. Discover the thrill of embracing the unknown and taking a leap of faith instead of hesitating on the fence. Don't settle for the easy way out - confront your fears head-on and embrace the exhilaration of taking that leap. Discover the incredible potential that lies within every failure - a wellspring of knowledge, a source of empowerment, and a stepping stone towards ultimate success.

Unlock the Power of Your Mindset

Unlock the power of your mind through the transformative practice of meditation. By taking action, you can liberate yourself from the shackles of fear and overcome the negative emotions that hold you back. Embrace the power to conquer your anxieties and free yourself from their grip.

Gain a fresh perspective

Unlock a new perspective and discover the art of personal growth. Embrace every setback as a precious gift; while undoubtedly challenging, it will serve as a valuable teacher, guiding you towards constant growth and transforming even the darkest moments into invaluable lessons.

Discover the power within you to conquer any fear. Fear may try to hold you back, but it's your choices that truly determine your path forward. Envision a life where your worries are effortlessly conquered, empowering you to reflect on your journey without the burden of regret. Seize control and banish the fear of failure from your narrative, ensuring a future free from remorse. Take control of your destiny.

Chapter 2

Unveiling the Secrets Behind Fear

Discover the myriad of factors that have the power to shape the onset of fear and unleash panic attacks in the human psyche. Introducing the remarkable factors that will captivate your attention:

Unleash the Power of the Evolutionary Survival Mechanism!

Experience the remarkable journey of life as nature ingeniously crafted the amygdalae, specialized organs designed to instinctively respond to danger signals. Experience heightened sensitivity to subtle cues, often triggered by past painful events. Discover the remarkable level of sensitivity found in the amygdalae of pets, a fact that has been extensively confirmed. Experience the extraordinary! In our cutting-edge experiments, a courageous rat fearlessly encounters a captivating combination of a startling foot shock and a mesmerizing sound.

Experience the power of audio as it ignites a surge of emotions within you. Brace yourself as the amygdalae, the very core of your instincts, respond to the spine-tingling sounds, unleashing a wave of fear indicators. Witness the extraordinary power of painful encounters as they forge the remarkable "speed dial (LTP) circuits," ready to spring into action at the mere sound of a related audio transmission. Experience the exquisite sensitivity of these organs to subtle cues. Discover the remarkable significance of the vertebrae, the very backbone of early fishes, amphibians, reptiles, birds, and mammals. These vital organs served as the diverse components of their intelligent brains.

Experience the spine-chilling world of Terror & Horror like never before!

Experience a surge of heightened emotions as dread, terror, and anxiety intertwine, creating an overwhelming sense of unease. Discover the fascinating world of risk assessment, where levels are intricately intertwined with the imminent danger that lies ahead. Experience a life free from worry, stress, and anxiety with our revolutionary solution. Say goodbye to the constant fear of harm in the foreseeable future. Experience a whirlwind of emotions with dread, terror, and stress that grip the very essence of the present moment. Experience the unparalleled intensity of terror and anxiety that can overpower even the strongest individuals, causing them to make choices that defy logic and reason. Discover the intriguing distinction between terror and horror. While terror may evoke a sense of impending danger, horror takes you on a chilling journey of discomfort and revulsion. Experience the power of fear, the emotion that ignites the amygdalae, allowing you to perceive the underlying essence of unsettling moments. Introducing the incredible amygdalae, the guardians of your memories. They tirelessly hold onto the images, words, and situations that come after the devastating experiences of damage, ridicule, interpersonal rejection, loss of loved ones, or career setbacks. They are here to ensure that nothing slips through the cracks. Discover the captivating phenomenon of Dread, where the mere presence of associated cues can ignite an overwhelming sense of fear, leaving the individual perplexed by its origin.

Experience the Power of Bodily Responses

Experience the incredible power of your body's natural response system. When your amygdalae detect signs of dread, your hypothalamus springs into action, effortlessly managing and balancing your reproductive, vegetative, endocrine, hormonal, visceral, and autonomic functions. Trust in the remarkable capabilities of your own body. Experience the incredible impact on your body as every breath, every bite, every beat of your heart, and every thought sets off a chain reaction of vitality and motion. Discover the fascinating connection between the amygdalae and dilated pupils. Uncover the hidden power of these indicators. Experience the incredible surge of brain activity with our revolutionary technology! Experience the hair-raising power of our products. Experience the incredible power of our revolutionary product that effectively reduces saliva, leaving your mouth area perfectly dry and comfortable. Experience the invigorating effects of our revolutionary product as it stimulates perspiration and effectively reduces pores and skin resistance. Discover a new level of freshness and vitality with our cutting-edge formula. Experience the ultimate comfort with our revolutionary product that not only maximizes your blood circulation, but also keeps your hands warm and cozy. Say goodbye to cold hands and hello to pure comfort. Experience the incredible power of our revolutionary indicators that enhance your breathing by accelerating inhalation and exhalation. These remarkable devices also widen bronchial pipes, allowing a greater influx of revitalizing air into your lungs. Experience the incredible benefits of tightening your abdominals, optimizing digestive function, and enhancing the efficiency of your excretory system. Experience the powerful effects of our revolutionary product as it works to naturally enhance the acidity in your stomach, potentially leading to a gentle cleansing effect.

Introducing the incredible signals of the adrenal gland! Brace yourself for a surge of cortisol, the ultimate stress-busting hormone. Prepare to witness a remarkable rise in glucose creation, providing your muscles and brain with the extra fuel they need to conquer any challenge that comes your way. Get ready to conquer stress like never before! Introducing the incredible indicators that work wonders for your body! These powerful signals boost blood circulation pressure, effortlessly release sugars into the bloodstream, and enhance the body's inclination for efficient bloodstream clotting. Experience the extraordinary benefits of these indicators today! Experience the incredible power of our signs as they work to boost red bloodstream cells in your anxious postural muscles, resulting in a remarkable reduction of hands and body tremors. Experience the incredible power of artery dilation, allowing for enhanced blood circulation to your skeletal muscles. Experience the remarkable effects of our revolutionary product as it optimizes and enhances your body's immune system, ensuring a seamless and efficient defense against diseases. Experience the power of the amygdalae as they orchestrate a symphony of biological events, enveloping your brain in a whirlwind of emotional turmoil, even before your conscious mind has a chance to assess the situation. Experience a world where prolonged fear signals are no longer triggered by real physical risk.

Experience the power of your instinctive brain as it skillfully navigates through interpersonal and professional challenges. By cleverly planning your body's response to freeze, flee, or defend itself, it overcomes obstacles with ease.

Discover the Incredible Long-Term Effects!

Discover the transformative power of a reliable escape route from risky business. Say goodbye to the insistent Dread signals of anxiety that can wreak havoc on your well-being. Experience a newfound sense of calm as your heart rate and blood circulation pressure gradually return to their natural state. Experience the detrimental effects of these conditions on your business. From heart palpitations to exhaustion, nausea to upper body pain, shortness of breath to stomach pains, and even headaches - these symptoms can hinder your productivity and overall well-being. Experience the power of escalating fear indicators that can trigger anxiety attacks, leaving you breathless and on edge. These attacks exhibit signs that can mimic the symptoms of cardiovascular attacks, heightening the intensity of your experience. Discover the remarkable connection between anxiety and various medical conditions that have been observed throughout the years. From arthritis to migraines, allergies to abdomen ulcers, and even thyroid disease, anxiety has been found to play a significant role in these health issues.

Discover the captivating world of Inherited, Acquired & The Unknown.

Introducing the incredible amygdala - the powerhouse behind your fear response! This remarkable part of your brain is responsible for triggering those crucial fear signals that propel you to take action and protect yourself from potential risks. It's like having a built-in alarm system that keeps you one step ahead of danger. So, next time you feel that rush of fear, remember that it's your amazing amygdala working tirelessly to keep you safe and sound. Introducing a product that effortlessly adapts to three distinct types of occasions. Discover the power of the first generation of inherited circuits as they delve into the depths of history to uncover and analyze past incidents of harm. Introducing the remarkable second band of neurons, diligently crafting LTP circuits that possess the extraordinary ability to ignite in the presence of identifying events, particularly those that are associated with less-than-pleasant experiences. Experience the thrilling conclusion of these captivating loops as they evoke a sense of trepidation, leaving the machine grappling with the profound implications of a crucial meeting.

Experience the allure of Historic Triggers

Discover the awe-inspiring power of nature's craftsmanship, as it meticulously constructs a memory sanctuary within the amygdala to store the recollection of perilous encounters. Discover the remarkable signs of these extraordinary moments, and witness the awe-inspiring power of the amygdala as it unleashes an overwhelming sensation of Dread. Introducing the common fears that plague us all: the fear of falling, the fear of suffocation in confined spaces, and the fear of encountering creepy crawlies like rats, cockroaches, or snakes. Discover the fascinating connection between stage fright and the primal instinct to capture the attention of predators. Unleash your inner performer and conquer your fear of public speaking. Experience the incredible power of the amygdala's worry reactions, which are often accompanied by the awe-inspiring startle response.

Introducing: Pain Experiences - Your Gateway to a World of Sensations!

Experience a remarkable transformation as the amygdala evolves to embrace a heightened perception of pain encounters over an extended period. Experience the transformative power of pain, a force that can be ignited by physical trauma, heart-wrenching conflicts, the absence of cherished companions, the void of social standing, or the sting of rejection in our relationships. Experience the profound impact of mirror neurons as they evoke a deep sense of empathy within us, allowing us to feel the pain of others as if it were our own. Experience the power of dread, triggered by the mere glimpse of a distressed countenance. Experience the profound depths of human emotion as individuals face the agonizing trials of failure, ridicule, and the heart-wrenching loss of loved ones. Experience the transformative power of overcoming childhood trauma. Imagine a world where loneliness no longer holds you back. Discover how to conquer your fears and embrace a life filled with connection and joy.

Discover the Enigmatic

Experience a world where fears of death, nuclear wars, terrorism, or even unsettling changes in work environments have no power over you. Break free from the shackles of these concerns and embrace a life filled with peace and tranquility. Discover the transformative power of recognizing the significance of a meeting, and say goodbye to fear. Discover Archy de Berker's insightful reviews on the captivating power of doubt in provoking terror. Discover the groundbreaking method of tracking stress levels in various topics. By precisely measuring changes in pupil diameter, our innovative approach taps into the release of the stress hormone "noradrenaline" in the mind. Discover the fascinating connection between pain and doubt as they both play pivotal roles in the realm of stress.

Discover the fascinating findings of a groundbreaking study. Participants in the experiment reported feeling significantly less Dread when they were aware that they would be facing pain, compared to those who were uncertain about the outcome. Uncover the intriguing relationship between knowledge and the perception of pain. Introducing a revolutionary solution for when you find yourself consumed by an overwhelming sense of Dread, with no clear path forward. Take control of your emotions by simply listing the problems that are causing you frustration. Discover the transformative power of confronting your deepest fears and liberating yourself from their grip. Embrace the opportunity to unravel the mysteries behind your anxieties and unlock a newfound sense of freedom and peace. Embrace the power of accepting doubt as an essential part of your environment, and watch as your fear diminishes.

Experience the Power of the Startle Response

Experience the power of fear as it ignites with the

electrifying startle response. Experience lightning-fast reflexes with your brain's rapid response time of just 20 milliseconds! According to the renowned Joseph Electronic LeDoux, this incredible feat is made possible through the primary amygdala Dread pathway. Prepare to be amazed by the speed and efficiency of your brain! Discover the extraordinary second path (300 milliseconds) that lies within the intricate reasoning procedures of the cortex, capable of triggering a sudden and overwhelming wave of Dread. Experience the power of the smallest stimuli as they ignite a surge of fear within you. Watch as your body reacts instinctively to even the slightest movements, noises, or images. Prepare to be startled by the intensity of your own response. Discover the innate power of the reflex, present from the moment of birth.

Experience the wonder of a newborn's reflexes! When a little one senses the slightest chance of falling, their delicate back arches and their tiny limbs flail with adorable enthusiasm. Skilled doctors carefully test these reflexes to ensure the development of the infant's nervous system. By simulating the sensation of falling, they gently allow the baby's head to drop ever so slightly. Witness the marvel of nature's instinctual responses in action! Experience the power of the amygdala's startle indicators as they ignite the sympathetic system, unleashing a surge of heightened psychological arousal. Experience the transformative power of cortical signs as they invigorate your parasympathetic system, gently alleviating mental tension. Experience the power of calmness as Unthinking Dread is effortlessly silenced by the rationality of the cortical indicators. Imagine the relief when you confidently discern that a coiled snake is nothing more than a harmless garden hose.

Revolutionize Your Response

Step into a world where physical risk was ever-present, where survival was a constant battle. But times have changed. Today, the relevance of that primitive world has diminished, as we navigate a safer and more secure environment. Unfortunately, when confronted with professional challenges, resorting to Dread reactions can be both inappropriate and detrimental. However, it is understandable to feel justified in the presence of a tiger. Experience a sense of ease and composure when faced with the possibility of being let go from your job. Experience the power of overcoming fear and unlock a world of financial freedom. Say goodbye to the burden of unpaid expenses and embrace a life of abundance. Let go of the tightness in your upper body and feel the weight lifted off your shoulders. It's time to break free from fear and start living your best life. Discover the solution to your problem with immediate clarity if it were within your reach. Discover the hidden dangers of anxiety caused by Dreads, which can have a profound impact on your overall well-being. Experience the peace of mind that comes with avoiding unexpected physical injury, while indulging in the irrelevance of Dread as a pet response. Discover the secret behind your fears - a primal neural response originating from the amygdala. But fear not, for there is a solution. Unlock the power of self-consciousness and silence the anxious whispers of your mind.

Discover the Power of Unconscious Avoidance

Experience the awe-inspiring instinct of animals as they face danger head-on. Witness the incredible power of their minds as they swiftly devise a strategic plan of action, perhaps even opting to gracefully slide under a rock and roll. Prepare to be amazed by nature's remarkable intelligence! Introducing Fear, the groundbreaking process that taps into the depths of your subconscious mind, relentlessly seeking out ingenious ways to escape from the clutches of pain. Discover the power of your impulsive decisions, driven by anxiety, as they shield you from the hidden pain you seek to evade. Experience the profound impact of various interpersonal emotions, such as sadness, disgust, contempt, guilt, and shame, that can trigger the sensation of pain. Discover the power of confidence and self-assurance by overcoming the fear of ridicule, empowering you to fully engage in meaningful conversations. Discover the captivating power of the Dread emotion, which has the potential to influence individuals to steer clear of challenging projects.

Introducing: Hormones - the key to unlocking your

body's full potential!

Experience an overwhelming sense of dread as the amygdalae, the fear center of the brain, react to specific sensory cues with heightened sensitivity. Experience the power of our revolutionary solution for patients battling post-traumatic stress symptoms. Unleash the potential to overcome unbearable Dread reactions, even to the point of fainting. Discover a new level of relief and reclaim control over your life. Discover the groundbreaking research by Richard Huganir, revealing the incredible power of manipulating targeted molecules that control synaptic plasticity in the amygdalae of our beloved pets. This revolutionary finding has the potential to eliminate the Dread response, offering a new ray of hope for pet owners everywhere. Introducing an extraordinary protein that has been uncovered, making its grand entrance in the amygdala of our beloved pets. These remarkable creatures have been expertly trained to respond to sounds that are linked to an unexpected foot surprise. Prepare to be amazed!

Introducing a remarkable molecule that, for a fleeting

moment, has the power to strengthen the fear circuits nestled within the intricate amygdalae. Experience the incredible results when our team of experts skillfully eliminate the protein, leading to a complete eradication of those haunting memories in the animals. Imagine a powerful combination of cutting-edge behavioural and pharmacological therapies, specifically designed to target those crucial molecular focuses. This groundbreaking approach holds the potential to revolutionize patient care and provide much-needed relief. Introducing groundbreaking research from the brilliant minds of Zurich scientists! Prepare to be amazed as they unveil their latest discovery: the incredible connection between the stress hormone oxytocin and sexual intercourse. But that's not all - brace yourself for the mind-blowing revelation that oxytocin also has the power to reduce amygdalae activity. Get ready to have your world turned upside down by this extraordinary scientific breakthrough!

Conquering Your Fears: A Guide to Overcoming Fear and Embracing Courage

Discover the power of personal awareness to effectively reduce the causes of Dread. Experience a newfound sense of calm as the rostral anterior cingulate cortex (rACC), the interest center of the mind, works its magic to reduce the intense activity in the amygdalae. Say goodbye to worries and embrace a more serene state of being. Experience the groundbreaking findings of Columbia University College researchers as they unveil the fascinating relationship between Dread stimuli and the remarkable role of rACC in regulating amygdalae activity. Witness the conscious recognition of Dread stimuli and the subsequent calming effect exerted by rACC. Prepare to be amazed by the intricate workings of the human brain! Discover the power of personal awareness and unlock the hidden potential of mind control methods to reveal the awe-inspiring global aftereffect of Dread. Discover the transformative power of fearlessness as a cultivated habit. Unlock the potential of personal awareness to cultivate a calm and tranquil mind.

Unlock the power of creative management with

unwavering alertness, leaving fear in the dust. Prepare to be captivated as fear becomes immobilized, and each breathtaking view reveals a thrilling and formidable allure. Introducing the ultimate solution for any daunting situation - the power of choice. When faced with life's challenges, you have not one, not two, but three incredible options at your disposal. Brace yourself for the possibilities that await! Take charge of the situation, steer clear of it, or embrace it as part of your life. Experience the power of a discreet assessment that will shape your reaction, all while acknowledging the lingering presence of potential threats. Experience the extraordinary sensation that arises when all fear is silenced. Unlock the power of success by harnessing the ability to carefully evaluate and embrace calculated risks.

Chapter 3

Discover the Intriguing World of Fear

Discover the power of fear as a profound motivator, making it crucial to understand when shifting your mindset. Introducing the power of overcoming fear! Imagine a world where concerns about change no longer hinder communication. Unlock the secret to success by understanding and addressing fear head-on, right from the start. Don't let fear hold you back - take charge and make your voice heard!

Introducing: Pain Solutions

Experience the undeniable power of pain. From the moment it touches your senses, you'll feel its relentless grip. And when pain reaches its peak, prepare yourself for an unparalleled level of intensity. Brace yourself for the sheer agony of extreme pain. It's a sensation that will leave you breathless, pushing the boundaries of your endurance. Embrace the excruciating journey Introducing the remarkable sensation of pain - a powerful mechanism designed to safeguard your precious body by prompting us to prioritize self-preservation. Experience the power of pain relief with our revolutionary message for pain projects. Discover the incredible benefits of minimizing excessive pain levels.

Experience the power of pain, transcending both the realms of the mind and the body. Experience the overwhelming burden of mental distress as it manifests in your very core, creating an intense sensation of pressure and stress. This emotional anguish can be just as excruciating as the physical pain inflicted upon your body. Experience fear like never before! Discover the fascinating way fear affects us, unraveling the mystery behind why we may feel fear.

Embrace the Power of Protecting What Matters Most

Experience a world of acquisitions as you journey through life, where each treasure is a testament to your dedication and hard work. Discover a world of possibilities with our collection of tangible goods and intangible experiences, including valuable connections and meaningful associations. Discover the captivating notion of relinquishing our hard-earned possessions, a concept that often evokes trepidation and has, intriguingly, given rise to a thriving insurance industry. Experience the profound emotion of loss, a natural consequence of the powerful bond we form with people and possessions. Through the process of attachment, we intertwine our sense of identity with these cherished elements, seamlessly extending ourselves. Experience the transformative power of reduction, where simplicity becomes the ultimate expression of personality. Embrace the essence of minimalism and leave behind the worries of extinction. Discover a world where less is truly more.

Experience the power of a stronger connection and unlock a heightened sense of anticipation. Feel the thrill as fear is amplified, taking you on an exhilarating journey. Discover the gripping fear that comes with the notion of parting ways with loved ones and close friends. Furthermore, it elucidates the very essence behind philosophies that advocate for a reduction in material abundance and even embracing a solitary existence as a hermit.

Introducing Non-gain Worries

Introducing the captivating concept of letting go: when you release what you currently possess, you open up a world of possibilities to acquire the very things you desire and anticipate. Introducing our incredible ability to foresee the imminent future, where our desires and aspirations take center stage. We have an unwavering knack for identifying the most coveted elements that propel us towards achieving our goals. Imagine the sheer dread that comes with the possibility of not acquiring the meticulously planned items we have set out to obtain. It fills us with an overwhelming sense of unease and trepidation.

Unlock the power to achieve your goals by mastering the art of controlling the world around you. Experience a sense of empowerment and security by achieving our goals. However, if we fall short, it's natural to feel a sense of vulnerability and apprehension. Experience the worry of missed opportunities, fueled by the fear of potential setbacks. Envision your deepest desires, only to be haunted by the looming sense of regret if you fail to take action.

Introducing: The Concern with Extinction

Discover the power of your identity, a fundamental need that is intricately intertwined with your sense of purpose and self-value. Experience the transformative power of embracing change. As things gradually diminish, a profound sense of reduction takes hold, leaving us with a newfound perspective on our place in the world. Witness how our perception of personality becomes beautifully fragmented, opening up endless possibilities for growth and self-discovery.

Discover the fascinating world of religions and their profound focus on life after death. Discover the profound significance of our identity when it is under threat, as we grapple with the pressing issue of extinction.

Discover the common concern of facing rejection from others. Expand your sense of connection by embracing everyone around you. Experience the transformative power of connection. When faced with rejection, our deep sense of self can be shattered, leaving us with an overwhelming sense of emptiness and solitude. Don't let loneliness consume you - discover the path to reconnection.

Embrace the Thrill of the Unknown

Introducing "The CIA Needs Model" - a revolutionary approach that addresses not one, but two crucial needs: a deep sense of identity and an unwavering sense of control. Discover the power of this groundbreaking model today. Experience the profound concern of potential extinction, where one's identity is at stake. Embrace the unease of relinquishing control and navigating the treacherous waters of uncertainty. Introducing the Fear of Non-Gain: the nagging worry that we may not reach our goals, leaving us to struggle in our pursuit of success.

Discover the underlying worry of losing control, as it dawns upon you that there are moments when individuals lack the ability to enhance their environment or influence the thoughts and actions of others. Achieving our goals requires navigating the unpredictable twists and turns of nature's whims and mastering the art of persuasion to sway others in our favor. Experience the overwhelming sense of helplessness when we find ourselves unable to accomplish a task. In those moments, it feels as if our world is spinning out of control.

Discover the intriguing world of individuals who possess their own unique aspirations, seemingly indifferent to our own desires, and perhaps even capable of skillfully influencing us. Unlock your full potential and conquer your personal goals like never before. Escape the clutches of manipulation and reclaim your autonomy. Don't let others devour your precious time and energy with their selfish demands. Take charge of your own needs and desires, and break free from the chains of people who seek to control you. Embrace your independence and live life on your own terms. Discover the remarkable ability of these individuals to achieve their goals through the sheer force of power, manifested in a multitude of captivating forms. Witness their unparalleled skill in the art of persuasion, as they effortlessly navigate the realms of influence. Experience the overwhelming sense of powerlessness and lack of control when influential individuals turn against us.

Discover the underlying concern of losing control, which may be intertwined with other anxieties like pain, decline, missed opportunities, or disappearance.

Embrace the Power of Overcoming Challenges

Unlock the power of control and take charge of your own destiny. Master the art of managing your emotions and acquire the essential skills needed to achieve your goals. Discover the thrilling notion that our deepest desires may elude us, sending shivers down our spines.

Introducing a concern that lingers in the back of our minds: the possibility of individuals responding impulsively, succumbing to anger or excitement, and engaging in actions that may haunt us in the future. Discover the detrimental impact of lacking self-control, a pressing concern that affects countless individuals.

Introducing a fear that resonates with many: the fear of failure. This fear often stems from a lack of skills, resulting in embarrassing mistakes and an inability to make a meaningful impact on others.

Introducing: Conditioned Fear - The Ultimate Thrill Experience!

Introducing a whole new perspective: Fear, redefined. It's not just any fear, but rather a fear that has been meticulously ingrained within us through conditioning. Experience the transformative power of fitness as it seamlessly bridges the gap between stimulus and response, igniting a renewed sense of vitality and energy. Experience the groundbreaking experiment of Pavlov, where a simple bell became the catalyst for an incredible discovery. Witness the power of sound as it effortlessly triggers the primal response of salivation in a dog. Prepare to be amazed by the remarkable connection between auditory stimulation and physiological reactions. Step into a world where a single sound can evoke a sensory experience like no other. Discover the fascinating connection between alarms and Fear, as recent research has revealed that even the mere association with electric shocks can activate this powerful emotion. Prepare to be captivated by the intriguing findings!

Discover the multitude of conditioned concerns that stem from childhood, where we mistakenly associated external stimuli with negative experiences. Discover the invaluable wisdom of embracing a healthy sense of caution when facing certain situations later in life. Discover the fascinating world of genetic anxieties, where our primal instincts collide with modern fears. Uncover the hidden depths of our psyche as we delve into the fearsome realms of spiders and snakes. Brace yourself for an exhilarating journey into the unknown! Step into a world where the mere sight of a single creature can send shivers down your spine. For ages, we have been conditioned to be wary of these furry companions, and the mere sight of them scurrying and writhing can trigger an intense and powerful Fear response.

Introducing: Phobia - Unveiling the 10 Most Common Worries That Plague Humanity

Introducing: Social Phobias - Conquer Your Fears and

Embrace Confidence!

Discover the fascinating world of interpersonal phobias, the most common and relatable form of fear.

Discover the incredible versatility and undeniable allure of these universal gems, known for their ability to capture the essence of excessive self-consciousness in any social setting.

Introducing a common concern that many individuals face: the fear of being judged. This fear can be so powerful that it leads them to avoid certain situations, such as eating in the presence of others.

Discover the shocking truth: 1 in 20 individuals suffer from the debilitating effects of interpersonal phobia.

Introducing Agoraphobia: Embrace the Thrill of Open Spaces!

Discover the hidden depths of agoraphobia, a fear that goes beyond public spaces. Experience the overwhelming panic that can grip you in the comfort of your own home, making even the simplest tasks seem insurmountable.

Discover the remarkable world of individuals with agoraphobia who courageously navigate their lives by skillfully avoiding specific places or venues.

Experience the thrill of Acrophobia: an exhilarating journey into the world of heights. Conquer your fears and embrace the adrenaline rush as you navigate towering heights with confidence. Don't let your concern with heights hold you back - let Acrophobia be your ticket to new heights of

Experience the thrill of fear like never before as you step onto the escalators at your neighborhood shopping center. These towering marvels of engineering are not for the faint of heart. Brace yourself for an adrenaline-pumping adventure that will leave you with a sense of vertigo like no other. Don't let fear hold you back - conquer your phobia and embrace the excitement that awaits you!

Experience the captivating sensation of Vertigo, a unique phenomenon that sets it apart from any ordinary phobia. Prepare to be enthralled by the exhilarating sense of dizziness that can envelop individuals. Experience the thrill of a lifetime with a cliff-top lookout or a towering building that will leave your mind spinning in awe.

Experience the exhilaration of soaring through the skies without a worry in the world with our exclusive Pteromerhanophobia solution. Say goodbye to your fear of flying and embrace the freedom of travel like never before.

Experience the allure of flying, even amidst the recent media frenzy surrounding air disasters. It's only natural to have concerns about plane crashes, but don't let that deter you from exploring the captivating world of aviation.

Discover the astonishing truth: amidst the staggering number of over 100,000 commercial plane tickets being sold worldwide each day, the chances of being struck by lightning are actually more substantial than the likelihood of perishing in a plane crash.

Experience the fear of enclosed spaces like never before with Claustrophobia! This gripping condition will have you on the edge of your seat as you navigate through tight spaces and face your deepest fears. Don't let claustrophobia hold you back - conquer it today!

Discover the hidden truth behind the fears of flying, where worries intertwine with concerns about confined spaces. Experience the overwhelming sensation of walls closing in with our Fear of Enclosed Spaces solution. Discover how our product can help those who feel trapped and confined, providing a sense of relief and freedom. Don't let the fear control your life any longer - take the first step towards liberation today.

Unlock the secrets of your fears with groundbreaking theories that propose a tantalizing genetic link to specific phobias. Dive into the fascinating world of dormant success mechanisms and discover the hidden forces that shape your deepest anxieties.

Experience the thrill of overcoming your fears with our revolutionary program, Entomophobia: Embrace the World of Insects. Discover a newfound appreciation for these fascinating creatures as we guide you through a journey of understanding and conquering your concerns. Don't let insects hold you back any longer -

Introducing the tiny creatures that crawl and occasionally leave a sting, it's no wonder that spiders and insects can evoke fear in many individuals.

Discover the undeniable importance of these incredible creatures as they serve as a vital link in the intricate web of the food chain. It's impossible to imagine a world without their invaluable presence.

Introducing Ophidiophobia: The Ultimate Guide to Overcoming Your Fear of Snakes

Discover the iconic words of Indiana Jones as he boldly declared, "I hate snakes," resonating with countless others who share his sentiment. Discover the widespread fear of all things long and venomous.

Discover the fascinating world of snakes, where a simple rule applies: give them space and they will graciously reciprocate. These enigmatic creatures possess a unique ability to coexist peacefully when left undisturbed.

Are you tired of feeling anxious around our furry friends? Say goodbye to your cynophobia and embrace a life filled with joy and companionship. Our expert team is here to help you overcome your fear of dogs and experience the love and loyalty that only a canine companion can provide. Don't

Introducing a fear of canines, a widely prevalent phobia that often affects children and door-to-door salespeople. Discover the power of overcoming your worries with an extraordinary animal encounter. Phobias can be challenging to conquer, especially when it comes to our furry friends. Canines have an uncanny ability to sense our fears, making it one of the most difficult phobias to overcome. But fear not, for there is hope!

Experience the thrill of a storm like never before with Astraphobia, the ultimate concern with storms. Get ready to be captivated by the power and beauty of nature as you embark on a journey of fear and fascination. Don't miss out on the electrifying experience of Astraphobia

Experience the exhilarating rush as the booming audio of thunder ignites your senses, causing your heart to race with anticipation.

Experience the awe-inspiring power of lightning, a force of nature that commands respect. While it is true that lightning has the potential to cause harm, rest assured that the likelihood of this occurring is incredibly rare. Your safety is our utmost priority.

Introducing Trypanophobia: Conquer Your Fear of Needles!

Discover the unsettling notion of a tiny, razor-sharp piece of steel lurking within your equipment, causing unease and discomfort. It's no wonder that needles evoke such a powerful aversion in many individuals. Discover the true value of needles as they bravely deliver life-saving vaccinations, facilitate crucial blood donations, and aid in the investigation of potential illnesses. They even have the power to create stunning works of art through the art of tattooing. Embrace the temporary discomfort for the greater good.

Chapter 4

Discover the Ultimate Guide to Overcoming Your Fear with These 14 Powerful Strategies!

As the New Year dawns, countless individuals contemplate the art of making resolutions to elevate themselves to new heights. Discover the unfortunate reality that many individuals, who excel at crafting resolutions, may ultimately fall short of their goals. Discover the secret to unlocking success and seizing opportunities, even in the face of overwhelming dread. Embrace the thrill of the unknown. For some, failure is a daunting prospect, while others are held back by the overwhelming potential of success. But imagine the possibilities if you could conquer both fears. Unlock your true potential and soar to new heights. Introducing a common obstacle that plagues countless individuals: worries. These pesky concerns have a knack for paralyzing even the most ambitious, hindering them from reaching their true potential and obtaining the success they so desire.

Discover the undeniable truth: refusing to take action is the ultimate recipe for failure. Introducing the ultimate solution to keep Dread from sabotaging your hustle this season. Discover the 14 powerful methods to triumph over fear and reach a stage where no obstacle can hinder your progress.

Embrace the Power of Fear and Embrace Your Journey. Introducing: Fear - Your Trusted Guardian. Discover the true power of this remarkable tool - neither inherently bad nor good, but a powerful instrument that empowers us to make smarter decisions. Embrace the power of dread! It's not meant to paralyze us, but to propel us into action. Discover the techniques that will unlock the results you desire and deserve. Embrace fear as a powerful tool for growth and let it guide your actions. But remember, don't let fear take the reins of your life.

Introducing the revolutionary approach: Don't settle for mere action, embrace the power of standing still! Experience the transformative effects of being present and taking a moment to observe. It's time to break free from the constant rush and discover the profound impact of standing there! Introducing the art of intentionality - a trait often overlooked in our fast-paced world. While we may be captivated by those who act swiftly, let us not forget the power of thoughtfulness, the beauty of ideation, and the importance of setting our own pace. Embrace the art of being deliberate and witness the magic unfold. Discover the unfortunate truth that countless individuals, who once experienced a promising beginning, have had their lives shattered or jeopardized due to the perils of haste. When faced with fear, it's important to pause and reflect. Instead of acting impulsively, take the time to explore your options and make a calculated decision. By doing so, you can ensure that you're making a wise and well-thought-out choice, rather than succumbing to the pressure of the moment.

Introducing: Name Worries - the ultimate solution for all your naming concerns! Discover the incredible strength that comes from simply acknowledging your fears. Unleash the power within by giving voice to your deepest fears, immortalize them on paper, or channel your thoughts towards them. Discover the power of overcoming your fears and watch them grow into something extraordinary. Discover the incredible power of facing your fears as they shrink away before your very eyes.

Unlock the power of foresight and embrace the art of thinking long term. As a savvy business owner, you may have concerns about meeting your next payroll with confidence. Looking ahead, let's explore your three-month perspective or envision the view three years down the line. When considering the long-term implications, it becomes clear that a quick fix won't solve your immediate problem. However, embracing this perspective can greatly benefit you in the long run. Experience a new level of clarity and unlock the perfect solution.

Stay ahead of the game by staying well-informed. Introducing the power of familiarity: the key to conquering your fears. Don't let your Dread be fueled by a lack of information. Empower yourself with the knowledge and insights necessary to analyze the problem based on concrete facts, not mere speculation.

Get ready, hone your skills, and engage in realistic scenarios. Introducing the all-time reigning champion of fears in the United States: presenting and public speaking. Discover the astonishing truth: in numerous studies, the act of speaking before a crowd ranks second only to death itself in terms of sheer terror. Are you feeling a sense of Dread when it comes to your performance in a specific activity? Don't worry, because I have the perfect solution for you. It's time to unleash your full potential by preparing, practicing, and engaging in some invigorating role-play. Say goodbye to those feelings of Dread and hello to a newfound confidence! Introducing Carmine Gallo, the brilliant author behind the acclaimed book Speak Like TED. In his captivating work, Gallo delves into the remarkable story of Dr. Jill Bolte-Taylor, a true TED sensation. With her awe-inspiring talk, which has garnered an astonishing 18 million views and counting, Dr. Bolte-Taylor has taken the stage over 200 times, leaving audiences spellbound.

Don't have enough time? No worries! According to Gallo, the presentation training sweet spot is a minimum of ten times. So, even with a busy schedule, you can still nail that presentation!

Harness the power of peer pressure. Have you ever experienced the thrill of taking a leap into the unknown? Picture this: standing on a towering bridge, your heart pounding with anticipation. The rush of adrenaline surges through your veins as you prepare to dive into the crystal-clear river below. What compels you to take this daring plunge? It's the contagious energy of your adventurous friends, urging you to embrace the exhilaration. Together, you create unforgettable memories that will forever ignite your spirit. Discover the incredible power of peer pressure, a force that can shape your world for the better or worse. Just like fear, its impact is determined by how it is harnessed. Surround yourself with a dynamic group of individuals who will propel you forward, helping you conquer the anxieties that have been holding you back from achieving your desires.

Experience the power of visualizing success. Experience the power of visualization as sports athletes envision the triumphant culmination of their hard work and dedication, replaying it in their minds countless times until it becomes a reality. Experience the power of mental mapping as your body effortlessly visualizes the path ahead, ensuring it stays on its pre-ordained route. Unlock the power of practice and pave your way to unparalleled success in any endeavor you set your sights on.

Experience a newfound sense of balance and harmony. Discover the incredible magnitude of our finished offer! Discover the offer that sends shivers down your spine. Discover the exhilarating journey of pursuing a quest, where success and failure intertwine with the values we hold dear. Sometimes, we become so captivated by the outcome that we lose sight of its connection to the bigger picture. Imagine the worst possible outcome. What could be more severe? Discover the power of truth. While it may be unsettling at times, you'll often realize that the fear of the unknown is far more daunting than the actual outcome you dread.

Discover the power of seeking assistance. Discover the thrill of facing your fears head-on. Could it be that the very thing you're afraid of is an opportunity for personal growth and empowerment? Embrace the challenge and consider taking it on solo. Discover the incredible potential of finding a dedicated coach or a supportive group to guide you through your journey. Discover the power of having your own personal instructor to guide and elevate your athletic performance. Unlock the power of knowledge with our exceptional team of educators, guiding students towards success. Discover the incredible power of friendship, where even those without firsthand knowledge can provide the essential support to conquer your deepest fears.

Discover the power of following others and uncover the secret formula for success. Are you blazing a trail that has yet to be traversed, or is it conceivable to tread in the footsteps of a trailblazer who has already achieved it? Discover the ultimate formula for achieving unparalleled success. Discover the possibilities of finding a book that delves into this very issue, or explore the potential of adapting a formulation from a different field to perfectly suit your needs.

Discover the power of a positive mindset. Introducing Brian Tracy's groundbreaking book: Be Unstoppable, Amazing, and Unafraid! Imagine the possibilities if you were guaranteed success in every endeavor. Picture a world where you have the power to make a difference. Now, ask yourself: what would you do differently? How would you seize every opportunity that comes your way? Embrace the limitless potential that awaits you and let your dreams become a reality. Experience a world of endless possibilities. Unlock your potential by exploring a wide range of options. Dare to try more and discover what you're truly capable of. Are you the type of person who perseveres long after others have thrown in the towel? Unlock the secret to success with a positive attitude that never quits. Those who possess unwavering positivity are the true champions, persisting where others falter. Embrace the power of a positive mindset and watch as success becomes your constant companion.

Embrace the art of adaptability and be ready to pivot at

a moment's notice. Introducing the timeless wisdom that has stood the test of time: "If at first you don't succeed, try, try again." Introducing the captivating phrase, "Insanity does a similar thing again and again and anticipating different results." Don't let fear hold you back from taking action again. Instead, take a closer look at why things didn't work out last time and explore new approaches before giving up completely. Remember, success often comes from perseverance and adaptability.

Discover the power of drawing inspiration from others. Discover a world where selflessness knows no bounds, where acts of kindness transcend personal limitations. Witness the incredible lengths people will go to for the sake of others, defying all expectations. Imagine the scene: Hyrum Smith, the brilliant co-founder of Franklin Covey, captivating his audience with a mesmerizing demonstration. In a moment of daring, he turns to a brave mother and poses a thrilling challenge. Picture this: a typical metallic "I beam" suspended high above the city, connecting two towering skyscrapers. Will she have the courage to cross this perilous path? The tension mounts as the crowd holds its breath... Introducing the resolute and unwavering response: "No, she wouldn't," she confidently declared. Imagine a scenario where he charmingly asks her if she would be willing to accomplish the task at hand for a whopping million-dollar reward. As if that wasn't enough, he playfully mentions the presence of a gentle breeze accompanied by the rhythmic sound of raindrops falling from the sky. She absolutely refused to budge. Imagine a scenario where he confidently assures her that he is taking care of her precious child in a secure location. However, he adds a sense of urgency by warning her that if she fails to arrive within a mere 10 seconds, he will reluctantly have to part ways with the child. Discover the true essence of her response amidst those challenging circumstances.

Chapter 5

Discover the Intriguing World of Phobias and Irrational Fears

Discover the fascinating world of human psychology, where even the bravest souls harbor their own irrational fears. Picture this: a shiver down your spine at the sight of two spiders or the anxiety that creeps in before your annual dental checkup. These fears, seemingly trivial, reveal the intricate workings of the human mind. Discover how these concerns can easily become a thing of the past for countless individuals. Introducing the remarkable phenomenon known as phobia: when anxieties reach such overwhelming levels that they unleash tremendous distress, impeding your ability to live a healthy and fulfilling life.

Discover the power of phobias - an extraordinary phenomenon where intense concern takes hold, even in the face of minimal or non-existent danger. Introducing the most common phobias and worries that haunt us all: closed-in places, levels, highway traveling, flying bugs, snakes, and needles. Brace yourself as we delve into the depths of these fears and anxieties that grip our souls. Discover the incredible power of the human mind as it can form phobias of practically anything. Discover the fascinating world of phobias, where fears can take root during the formative years of childhood or emerge later in life.

Discover the perplexing world of phobias, where the mind's logic battles against the overwhelming power of fear. Despite the undeniable awareness of the irrationality, one's emotions remain stubbornly beyond control. Discover the incredible power that even the mere thought of a feared object or situation can have over your stress levels. Introducing the revolutionary experience: the moment you encounter it, your senses are instantly consumed by an automated wave of fear and overwhelming terror. Brace yourself for the ultimate thrill! Discover the power of knowledge that is so captivating, it may drive you to extraordinary measures to evade it, inconveniencing yourself or even transforming your entire way of life. Imagine this: You're faced with a golden opportunity, a job offer that could potentially bring you great success. But here's the catch - the office is located on a higher floor, and you have to take the elevator to get there. Now, if you happen to suffer from claustrophobia, this seemingly simple task can quickly turn into a nightmare. The fear of enclosed spaces can overpower your rational thinking, causing you to pass up on a potentially lucrative opportunity. Don't let claustrophobia hold you back from reaching your full potential. Explore ways to conquer your fears and unlock a world of possibilities. Discover the ultimate solution for conquering your fear of heights. Imagine never having to detour an extra 20 miles just to avoid a towering bridge. With our revolutionary program, you'll gain the confidence to face any altitude with ease. Say goodbye to anxiety and hello to a world of limitless possibilities. Take the first step towards freedom today!

Unlocking the power to conquer your phobia begins with a deep understanding of its inner workings. Discover the undeniable importance of understanding that phobias are a perfectly normal part of life. Discover the truth: Having a phobia doesn't mean you're crazy! In fact, it's important to understand that phobias can be effectively treated. Unlock the power within you to conquer stress, anxiety, and fear, and embark on a life of fulfillment and joy. No matter how overwhelming it may appear, you have the ability to take control and shape the life you desire.

Discover Jane's captivating journey through the skies.

Experience the thrill of soaring through the skies with Jane, as she conquers her fear of flying. Regrettably, she finds herself having to embark on multiple journeys for work, each one exacting a dreadful toll on her well-being. Experience the anticipation like never before. Feel the excitement build up inside her, creating a delightful knot in her tummy. Despite the nerves, there's an undeniable thrill that lingers, adding an extra touch of magic to each trip. Embrace the journey and let the adventure unfold. Experience the thrill of anticipation as she awakens on the day of her airline flight, a sense of excitement coursing through her veins. Experience the thrill as she steps onto the plane. Her heart races, her head feels light, and she starts to breathe rapidly. Experience the ultimate decline with each and every journey.

Jane's deep-seated fear of flying has reached such an extreme level that she has made the courageous decision to inform her manager that she can only commit to attending events and locations that are within a reasonable driving distance. Discover the story of Jane, a dedicated employee whose employer was less than thrilled with recent events. Now, Jane finds herself unsure of what lies ahead in her career. Experience the gripping fear of potential demotion or even the terrifying possibility of losing one's job entirely. Discover the true power of self-belief, surpassing any fear of boarding another plane.

Discover the distinction between "normal fears" and phobias or what some may call "irrational fears".

Embrace the power of Fear in perilous situations, for it is not only normal but also advantageous. Experience the power of terror as it serves to protect, activating your body's automated "fight-or-flight" response. Experience the power of instant notification and heightened awareness. With our cutting-edge technology, both your body and mind will be primed and prepared to take action. React swiftly and shield yourself from any potential threats with ease. Discover the fascinating world of phobias, where the threat is nothing more than a figment of the imagination or blown out of proportion. Imagine this scenario: you find yourself face to face with a snarling Doberman. It's only natural to feel a twinge of hesitation. However, let's consider a different situation. Picture yourself encountering a friendly poodle, happily wagging its tail while being held on a leash. Now, it would be completely irrational to be terrified of this adorable poodle, wouldn't it? Unless, of course, you happen to have a puppy phobia.

Discover the Distinction: Fear vs. Phobia

Introducing the all-new, revolutionary

Experience the thrill of normal anxiety like never before!

Experience the thrill of soaring through the skies, even in the face of turbulence or stormy weather. Don't let anxiety hold you back from the exhilaration of flight. Experience the joy of attending your best friend's island wedding without the hassle of travel. Feel the exhilaration of butterflies fluttering in your stomach as you gaze down from the pinnacle of a towering skyscraper or ascend a lofty ladder. Experience the thrill of turning down congratulations, all while being situated on the prestigious 10th floor of a magnificent office building.

Experience a slight sense of unease when receiving a shot or having your blood drawn. Discover the freedom of embracing essential procedures and doctor's checkups without fear, liberating yourself from the grip of needle phobia.

Introducing: Normal Fears in Children!

Discover the fascinating world of childhood fears, where natural instincts intertwine with specific developmental stages. Introducing the perfect solution for small children who fear the dark - the nightlight! Say goodbye to restless nights and hello to peaceful sleep with this must-have accessory. Discover the truth behind their fears. Experience the incredible transformation as they naturally outgrow their fears with age.

Introducing the next generation of childhood fears that are not only widespread but also considered completely normal:

Introducing the Sensory Sensations Collection! Designed to captivate and engage your little one's senses, our range of products is perfect for babies and toddlers aged 0-2 years. From the thrilling sounds of loud noises to the excitement of meeting new strangers, our collection embraces the challenges of separation from parents and the awe-inspiring world of large objects. Discover a world of sensory exploration with our carefully crafted products!

Discover a world of imagination with our carefully curated collection for children aged 3-6 years. From friendly ghosts to mysterious monsters, we have everything to spark their creativity and conquer their fears. Let them explore the wonders of the dark, embrace the thrill of sleeping alone, and conquer their fear of unusual noises. Our selection is designed to inspire and entertain, making every moment a magical adventure.

Introducing our exclusive range of fears for the age group of 7-16 years! Brace yourself for a thrilling experience as we dive into the world of more realistic fears. From the fear of injury and illness to the anxiety surrounding school performance and the loss of life, we've got it all covered. And that's not all - prepare to be captivated by the fear of natural disasters that will leave you on the edge of your seat. Get ready to embark on an unforgettable journey through the depths of these gripping fears!

Discover peace of mind knowing that if your child's Fear is not disrupting their daily life or causing excessive distress, there is no need for unnecessary worry. Introducing the solution to your child's worries! If those worries are getting in the way of their social life, academic success, or much-needed rest, it's time to consider the expertise of a skilled child therapist.

Discover the Fascinating World of Phobias and Fears

Introducing the revolutionary "FearShield" - the ultimate solution for those moments when fear takes hold. Say goodbye to the days of hiding behind your hands! With FearShield, you can confidently face any challenge that comes your way. Don't let

Discover the fascinating world of phobias and fears, where four distinct types await your exploration:

Introducing the all-new, highly anticipated

1.Discover the fascinating world of animal phobias, where fears of snakes, spiders, rodents, and dogs take center stage.

2 Environment Phobias - Your Ultimate Concerns Unveiled!

3. situational phobias, the fears that arise from specific situations. Experience the thrill of enclosed spaces with claustrophobia, embark on a journey of fear with flying and traveling, and brace yourself for the adrenaline rush of tunnels and bridges.

4. the Blood-Injection-Injury phobia, where fears of blood, injury, illness, needles, and surgical procedures take center stage.

Discover a world of phobias that defy the ordinary and transcend the common categories. Introducing a collection of worries that will leave you breathless. Experience the thrill of concerns with choking, the suspense of obtaining a disease like malignancy, and the spine-tingling fear of clowns. Brace yourself for an unforgettable journey into the depths of your deepest fears. Discover a world of uncommon phobias that defy categorization:

Introducing social phobia, the ultimate fear of interpersonal situations where the mere thought of being judged or feeling ashamed sends shivers down your spine. Discover the transformative power of overcoming interpersonal phobia. Unleash your true potential by conquering self-consciousness and fear of humiliation. Embrace a life free from the shackles of social anxiety. Discover the secret to unlocking your true confidence and embracing every interpersonal situation with ease.

Don't let the fear of judgment hold you back from enjoying life to the fullest.

Introducing the all-too-common phobia: fear of general public speaking. This interpersonal phobia is something many individuals can relate to. Discover the multitude of concerns that come hand in hand with interpersonal phobia. From the anxiety of eating or consuming in public, to the fear of speaking with strangers, taking examinations, mingling at a celebration, or even being called on in class, this condition can truly impact various aspects of your life.

Introducing Agoraphobia: The Fear of Open Spaces Discover the fascinating world of Agoraphobia, a condition that was once believed to be limited to open public places and vast open spaces. However, recent research has shed new light on this complex disorder, revealing its close connection to anxiety attacks.

Introducing a solution for those who fear the dreaded anxiety attack: a feeling of unease that arises when faced with potentially awkward or embarrassing situations. Imagine a world where you effortlessly steer clear of bustling stores and packed concert halls. Experience the power to safeguard against all modes of transportation - from cars and planes to subways and more. Experience the ultimate sense of security within the comfort of your own home, even in the most challenging circumstances.

Discover the Telltale Signs and Symptoms of Phobias

Experience the wide spectrum of symptoms that a phobia can unleash, from a mere sense of unease to an overwhelming anxiety attack. Experience the power of proximity. The closer you venture towards the very essence of your fears, the more intense your Fear will become. Embrace the thrill of pushing your limits and watch as your courage soars to new heights. Experience the heightened intensity of fear when escape seems impossible.

Experience the undeniable physical manifestations of a phobia, which may include:

- Experience the sensation of effortless breathing.

- Experience the exhilaration of a race or feel the pulsating rhythm of your heart.

- Experience the ultimate relief from upper body pain or tightness.

- Experience the sensation of trembling or shaking like never before!

- Experience a world of dizziness and light-headedness.

- Experience the sensation of a churning stomach like never before!

- Experience the invigorating sensation of hot or cool flashes, accompanied by delightful tingling sensations.

- Experience the invigorating sensation of perspiration.

- Experience the power of the mind with the psychological symptoms of a phobia:

- Experience the overwhelming power of anxiety

and panic.

- Escape to the ultimate freedom.

- Experience a sense of being "unreal" or disconnected from your own self.

- Experience a sense of unease about losing control or feeling overwhelmed.

- Experience the sensation of being on the brink of transcendence.

- Discover the profound awareness of recognizing your tendency to overreact, while simultaneously experiencing a sense of helplessness in managing your own fear.

- Discover the telltale signs of Blood-injection-injury Phobia

- Discover the unique symptoms that set blood-injection-injury phobia apart from other phobias. Experience a rush of emotions when confronted with the sight of the bloodstream or a needle - a potent mix of Fear and disgust.

Experience the exhilaration of a racing heart as you embark on a journey through the world of phobias. Experience the thrill like no other! Unlike any other phobias, brace yourself for an exhilarating acceleration that will leave you breathless. But that's not all - prepare for a heart-pounding adventure as your blood circulation pressure takes an instant plunge, causing a rush of sensations like nausea, dizziness, and even fainting. Get ready to push your limits and embrace the adrenaline rush! Experience the unique phenomenon of fainting exclusively in the blood-injection-injury phobia, where concern with fainting is a hallmark feature.

Discover the Perfect Time to Seek Assistance for Phobias and Fears

Discover the fascinating world of phobias, where normalcy meets intrigue. While these fears may not always bring about substantial distress or disrupt your daily life, they still hold a captivating power over the human psyche. Imagine living in a city where the chances of encountering a snake are incredibly slim. With this ideal scenario, even if you have a deep-rooted fear of snakes, it would have absolutely no impact on your daily life. No more worries, no more anxieties. Embrace a snake-phobia-free existence! Introducing an alternative perspective: imagine living in a sprawling metropolis, but if you happen to have an intense fear of crowded places, this could pose quite a challenge.

If your phobia has minimal impact on your daily life, there's no need to worry. Are you tired of letting your phobia control your life? Don't let fear hold you back from enjoying the things you love. It's time to take action and get the help you need to overcome your phobia. Don't let it inhibit your normal working or prevent you from doing the things you truly enjoy. Take the first step towards a life free from fear and get the support you deserve.

Unlock a world of possibilities by exploring treatment options for your phobia. Discover the freedom and peace of mind that awaits you. Take the first step towards conquering your fears and living life to the fullest. Don't let your phobia hold you back any longer. Embrace the opportunity for growth and transformation. Seek treatment today

Experience the overwhelming power of fear and panic like never before with our revolutionary product. Prepare to be taken to new heights of intensity as you encounter extreme and disabling emotions that will leave you breathless.

Discover how your Fear can be transformed into a powerful force. Recognize the excessive and unreasonable nature of your Fear, and take the first step towards reclaiming control over your life.

Discover the freedom of overcoming your phobia and reclaiming control over your life. Say goodbye to avoiding situations and places that hold you back, and embrace a future filled with confidence and fearlessness.

Introducing the groundbreaking solution to your avoidance struggles! Say goodbye to inhibitions and distress that disrupt your normal routine. Experience a life free from the burdens of avoidance with our revolutionary product.

Introducing the remarkable phobia that has persisted for a minimum of six months.

Conquer Your Phobia: Overcoming Fear with Confidence

Discover the powerful combination of self-help strategies and therapy, proven to effectively conquer even the most challenging phobias. Discover the perfect solution tailored just for you, based on crucial factors such as the level of intensity of your phobia, your utilization of professional treatment, and the amount of support you require.

Discover the transformative power of self-help and unlock your true potential. Embrace the journey of personal growth and embark on a path towards success and fulfillment. Give yourself the gift of self-improvement and experience the incredible benefits it can bring. Don't hesitate, take the leap and see how self-help can truly make a difference in your life. Unlock your true potential and experience the empowering feeling of being in control. Elevate yourself to new heights and watch as your fears and anxieties fade away. Discover the power of seeking additional support if your phobia is causing severe distress, anxiety attacks, or overwhelming anxiousness. Don't let fear hold you back - take control of your life today.

Discover the remarkable history of phobia therapy. Experience the exceptional performance and rapid results of our product. In as little as two to four classes, you'll witness its remarkable effectiveness. Discover the power of support that goes beyond the confines of a specialist therapist. Experience the incredible power of having someone by your side, ready to hold your hands or stand by your side as you confront your worries. This simple act of support can make a world of difference in your journey.

Discover the Power of Phobia Self-help!

Face Your Concerns, One Step at a Time!

Experience the thrill of a lifetime with our heart-pounding "Scared Man in an Elevator" adventure! Brace yourself as you step into the elevator, where suspense and excitement await. Feel the adrenaline rush as the elevator ascends, taking you on a journey filled with unexpected twists and

Discover the innate human instinct to steer clear of situations that evoke fear. Discover the key to conquering phobias: facing your anxieties head-on. Discover the power of facing your fears head-on. While it may be tempting to avoid them, doing so only hinders your personal growth and prevents you from realizing that your phobia is not as daunting as it seems. Embrace the opportunity to overcome your fears and unlock a world of possibilities. Discover the invaluable chance to master the art of managing your worries and gain full control over any problem that comes your way. Experience the spine-chilling intensity as this phobia takes hold, growing ever more daunting within the depths of your mind.

Discover the power of conquering your phobia with a tried and true method: gradual and controlled exposure to your deepest fears. By facing your fears head-on in a secure environment, you can unlock the path to freedom and overcome any obstacle that stands in your way. Discover the secrets to effortlessly banishing stress, anxiety, and fear during this transformative publicity process. Experience the transformative power of facing your Fear head-on. Discover that the worst-case scenario is nothing more than a figment of your imagination. Rest assured, you won't meet your demise or lose control. With each encounter, watch your confidence soar and your sense of control strengthen. Experience the incredible transformation as the phobia's power begins to diminish.

Discover the key to success by embarking on a journey that begins with a challenge within your grasp. Take confident strides as you ascend the "Fear ladder," honing your self-assurance and mastering invaluable coping skills along the way.

Create an organized and efficient list

Experience the spine-chilling tales that revolve around your deepest fears. Delve into a bone-chilling summary of the hair-raising situations that are intricately intertwined with your phobia. Are you afraid of flying? Well, fear no more! We have got you covered with a comprehensive checklist to ease your worries. From reserving your ticket to packing your suitcase, from the excitement of driving to the airport terminal to witnessing the majestic planes take off and land, from going through the necessary security procedures to finally boarding the flight of your dreams, and not to forget, the soothing voice of the flight attendant as they present the essential safety instructions. Sit back, relax, and let us guide you through this incredible journey.

Construct Your Fear Ladder

Discover the thrill of organizing your list in a spine-tingling fashion, from the least hair-raising to the most bone-chilling. Prepare to embark on an exhilarating journey as you take your first step on the ladder of excitement. Feel a delightful sense of anticipation, without any overwhelming fear that might hinder your exploration. Are you ready to conquer the ladder? Let's start by envisioning your objectives - perhaps you dream of fearlessly embracing your furry friends without a hint of panic. Now, let's break it down into manageable steps, each one bringing you closer to that ultimate goal.

Ascend the ladder to success

Experience the power of starting small and taking one step at a time. Embrace the first rung on the ladder and allow yourself to feel at ease before moving forward. Your journey begins with finding comfort in the present moment. Experience the power of perseverance by staying in the midst of challenges until your nerves fade away. Experience the transformative power of facing your fears head-on. By immersing yourself in the very thing that scares you, you will gradually become desensitized to it. As a result, the anxiety and stress that once plagued you will diminish, leaving you more confident and resilient for future encounters. Experience the exhilaration of conquering each step in a series of individual events, effortlessly gliding past any stress that may arise. With each successful ascent, you'll gain the confidence to seamlessly transition to the next exciting challenge that awaits. Introducing the ultimate solution for tackling overwhelming tasks: the power of breaking it down. Don't let the enormity of a step hold you back - simply break it into smaller, more manageable steps. And if that's not enough, take it slow and steady. Remember, progress is progress, no matter the pace.

Master your skills with relentless practice.

Experience the power of consistent practice and witness your progress soar to new heights. The secret lies in the frequency of your dedication - the more you commit, the faster you'll see remarkable improvement. Unlock your potential and embrace the journey of continuous growth. But wait, don't rush. Experience the thrill of progress at a pace that suits your comfort level, ensuring you never feel overwhelmed. Experience the temporary discomfort and stress as you confront your concerns, knowing that these emotions will soon dissipate. Experience the transformative power of perseverance as the overwhelming panic gradually dissipates.

Discover the secrets to achieving rapid relaxation

Experience the unsettling grip of fear and anxiety as your heart races and a suffocating sensation takes hold. Experience the overwhelming power of these physical sensations, as they grip you with fear and leave you trembling. The sheer distress caused by your phobia amplifies the intensity, making it an even more daunting experience. Discover the power of mastering the art of rapid relaxation. Unlock a newfound sense of confidence as you build resilience to discomfort and confront your fears head-on.

Experience the transformative power of a simple yet effective yoga breathing exercise. Experience the transformative power of deep, calming breaths. In moments of stress, it's common to find yourself caught in a cycle of rapid, shallow breaths, also known as hyperventilating. This only intensifies the overwhelming emotions of anxiety. Take control of your well-being by embracing the practice of deep, intentional breathing. Discover the profound impact it can have on your state of mind. Breathe your way to a calmer state of mind.

Experience the transformative power of deep, belly-filling breaths. By consciously inhaling and exhaling from the depths of your stomach, you can effortlessly reverse those pesky physical sensations that come with anxiety, breathlessness, and stress. Embrace a sense of tranquility and abundance as you effortlessly tap into the limitless well of calm that resides within you. Unleash your full potential by dedicating yourself to intense practice sessions, even during moments of tranquility. Embrace the challenge and push yourself to become intimately acquainted and effortlessly at ease with the exercise.

Experience the ultimate comfort as you sit or stand with perfect posture. Feel the support of your back as it remains in a straight and aligned position. Experience the power of balance by placing one hand gently on your upper body, while the other finds its place on your belly.

Experience the calming sensation as you gently inhale through your nostrils, savoring each deliberate breath. Experience the gentle rise of your abdomen as you place your hands on it. Experience the effortless grace of a perfectly executed motion as your upper body remains steady and composed, with minimal movement of the hands.

Experience the power of breath control with our revolutionary technique. Take a moment to savor the sensation as you hold your breath for a count of seven.

Experience the ultimate release as you gently exhale through your mouth, effortlessly pushing out every last bit of air. Feel the power of your stomach muscles engaging, creating a sense of strength and control. Experience the gentle rhythm of your breath as the hands on your tummy gracefully sway with each exhale, while your other hands remain still, allowing you to find a sense of calm and balance.

Experience the rejuvenating power of deep breaths as you embark on a journey towards ultimate relaxation and inner peace. Allow yourself to inhale deeply, embracing the tranquility that fills your being. Repeat this invigorating routine, each breath bringing you closer to a state of complete serenity and centeredness.

Discover the transformative power of this invigorating yoga breathing technique. Dedicate just 5 minutes, twice a day, to unlock a world of inner peace and vitality. Embrace the harmony that comes from connecting with your breath and experience the profound benefits that await you. Discover the power of this incredible method and unlock a world of possibilities. Once you become truly at ease with its techniques, you'll be able to harness its potential to conquer your deepest fears and overcome even the most challenging situations. Embrace the freedom and confidence that await you as you face your phobias head-on and navigate through the most stress-filled moments with ease.

Experience the world through your senses.

Experience the ultimate audio immersion with our cutting-edge headphones for men. Elevate your music listening experience to new heights and indulge in crystal-clear sound quality that will transport you to another world. Whether you're a

Discover the ultimate solution to conquer stress and

anxiety with ease and reliability. Engage your senses in a symphony of sight, sound, taste, smell, and touch. Experience the power of motion as you embark on a journey towards tranquility. Discover the power of individuality! Embrace the art of experimentation to uncover the most effective strategies tailored just for you.

Experience the joy of movement with our incredible range of walks and leaps. Gently extend your body as you explore the world around you. Experience the incredible power of dance, drumming, and operating to effortlessly melt away stress and anxiety.

Indulge your senses with the power of sight. Feast your eyes on the things that bring you joy and tranquility. Immerse yourself in the beauty of a breathtaking view, reminisce with cherished family photos, or let adorable kitty pictures on the web bring a smile to your face.

Introducing the perfect solution for a peaceful ambiance - Sound! Immerse yourself in the soothing melodies of calming music, let your voice soar as you sing your favorite melody, or unleash your inner rhythm with the enchanting beats of a drum. Experience the power of sound to create a serene atmosphere like never before. Indulge in the soothing sensations of nature's beauty, whether experienced firsthand or captured on film: the rhythmic ebb and flow of the sea waves, the gentle caress of the wind through the trees, and the melodious symphony of birdsong.

Experience the delightful aromas that surround you. Indulge in the gentle fragrance of scented candles, immerse yourself in the natural scents of a vibrant garden, and inhale the pure, refreshing oxygen. Enhance your senses by spritzing on your favorite perfume, creating an aura of elegance and allure.

Indulge in the exquisite pleasure of savoring every bite of your favorite treat, allowing its delightful flavor to unfold gradually with each slow and deliberate nibble. Indulge in the exquisite pleasure of sipping on a cup of all-natural tea or savor the invigorating burst of flavor from a refreshing stick of mint gum or your beloved hard candy.

Indulge in the luxurious experience of a soothing hand or neck massage therapy. Treat yourself to the ultimate relaxation and rejuvenation with our expert touch. Experience the heartwarming embrace of a beloved family pet. Indulge in the luxurious embrace of a velvety blanket. Experience the ultimate relaxation as you take a seat outside, basking in the refreshing cool airflow.

Discover the transformative power of meditation for ultimate anxiety and stress relief.

Discover the transformative power of yoga, a remarkable relaxation technique that not only alleviates anxiety but also has the potential to reshape the very structure of your brain. Experience the transformative power of yoga through regular practice. Discover how it can elevate your emotional well-being, fostering a deep sense of serenity within. By engaging the region of the mind that governs tranquility, yoga becomes a powerful tool to preemptively combat fear and stress. Embrace the calm before the storm with the help of yoga.

Mastering the art of conquering your phobia: Expert

tips on managing negative thoughts

Discover the fascinating world of phobias, where your imagination can run wild. Experience the thrill of overestimating the intensity of your fears and underestimating your own incredible strength to overcome them. Don't miss out on the exhilarating journey of conquering your deepest anxieties. Introducing the revolutionary solution to combat those pesky stress-induced thoughts and energy phobias! Say goodbye to negativity and unrealistic expectations with our groundbreaking approach. Discover the transformative power of capturing the toxic thoughts that arise when confronted with your deepest fears. By doing so, you can begin to challenge and overcome these unproductive patterns of thinking. Introducing a collection of thoughts that frequently fall into the following categories:

Unlock the secrets of your future with our captivating "Fortune-telling" experience.

Imagine the sheer terror of witnessing a bridge on the

verge of collapse. The heart-pounding fear that courses through your veins as you contemplate the possibility of making a complete fool of yourself. The overwhelming anxiety that grips you when the elevator doors start to close. These are just a few examples of the intense emotions that can consume us in moments of uncertainty.

Introducing the powerful concept of overgeneralization!

Experience the thrill of a lifetime with our exhilarating rides. Picture this: you're soaring through the air, feeling the wind rush past you, when suddenly... you faint. That's right, our rides are so intense, they'll leave you breathless. Don't miss out on the ultimate adrenaline rush - book your adventure today! Experience the thrill of a lifetime with heart-pounding excitement! Feel the adrenaline rush as you face your fears head-on. Witness the incredible power of a pit bull terrier as it lunges towards you. Brace yourself for the ultimate challenge, where fainting is not an option. Are you ready to conquer your fears and take another shot? Introducing the untamed world of canines - a realm where danger lurks at every turn. Brace yourself for an exhilarating journey through the wild side of nature.

Introducing Catastrophizing: The Art of Amplifying Worries

Experience the thrill of soaring through the skies as the captain fearlessly guides us through the exhilarating turbulence ahead. Experience the thrill of a lifetime as you witness the heart-pounding action of a plane soaring through the sky!" Witness the power of human connection," I thought to myself as the person beside me emitted a gentle cough. Discover the possibility of it being the notorious swine flu. Prepare yourself for an impending illness.

Chapter 6

Discover the secrets to conquering anxiety and stress!

Experience the power of panic as it unveils reliable indicators of response in times of emergencies. Imagine being caught in a blazing fireplace or facing an unexpected attack. Panic becomes your ally, guiding you towards swift action and survival. Experience the transformative power of our product as it effortlessly tackles not only high-pressure situations like exams, presentations, and public speaking, but also everyday events such as starting a new job, going on a date, or attending a party. Prepare to face any challenge with confidence and ease. Experience the innate instinct to protect yourself from potential dangers, whether they are perceived or genuine.

Introducing Stress: Unveiling the Intriguing World of Fear

Experience the relentless grip of anxiety and stress as they linger, refusing to release their hold. These unwelcome companions can persist, trapping you in their clutches for an extended period of time. Experience the overwhelming impact they can have on your daily life - from disrupting your eating and sleeping patterns, to hindering your ability to focus and enjoy simple pleasures. Don't let them hold you back from going out, pursuing your passions, or excelling in your professional or academic pursuits. Don't let this hold you back from pursuing the things you desire or need to accomplish.

Discover how to conquer your fears and embrace new opportunities with confidence. Don't let fear hold you back from living your best life. Take control and face your fears head-on, knowing that you have the power to overcome any challenge that comes your way. Breaking free from the monotony of your routine can be quite challenging, but fear not! There are numerous effective strategies to help you conquer this daunting task. Discover the secrets to conquering fear and reclaiming control over your life. Learn how to diminish feelings of fear and develop effective coping strategies that will empower you to live life to the fullest.

Discover the Power Within: Conquer Your Fears!

Experience a multitude of heart-pounding moments that will send shivers down your spine. Embrace the power of fear, for it can be your greatest ally in the face of danger. Take, for instance, the fear of fires. By acknowledging and respecting this fear, you are equipping yourself with the necessary caution and vigilance to ensure your safety. Remember, it is through our fears that we find the strength to protect ourselves. Embrace the power of ambition and strive for prosperity, for it is the driving force that propels you forward. However, tread carefully, for the overwhelming fear of failure can hinder your path to success.

Discover the fascinating ways in which individuals experience fear and navigate through it. The unique combination of what triggers your fears and your personal coping mechanisms make for a truly individualized experience. Discovering the root cause of your fears is the crucial first step towards conquering them.

Discover the secrets to effectively managing and reducing stress! Introducing our exclusive pocket guide, now available for free download! Discover the ultimate collection of 101 expert tips that will revolutionize your life. Don't miss out on this invaluable resource!

Discover the Reasons Behind Your Anxiety

Experience the power of understanding stress. Just like fear, nervousness is a form of stress. So, the characteristics we've discussed for fear also hold true for stress. Discover the fascinating connection between these two emotions.

Introducing the remarkable concept of 'anxiety' - a powerful word that captures the essence of worry and the relentless persistence of fear over time. Discover the power of anticipation. This incredible tool is utilized to address concerns that lie in the realm of the future, rather than focusing solely on the present moment. Embrace the possibilities that lie ahead and unlock a world of potential.

Experience the power of panic, a phrase that resonates with medical researchers as they delve into the depths of persistent fear. Experience the remarkable similarity between the techniques you feel when you're filled with fear and overwhelmed by stress. Discover how these two emotions share a common thread, as they both evoke a powerful and undeniable sensation.

Experience the Unsettling Sensations of Anxiety and Stress

Experience the incredible power of your brain and body when faced with fear or intense anxiety. Witness the remarkable speed at which they work to protect and guide you. Discover the exciting possibilities that await:

Experience the exhilaration of a heart that beats with lightning speed, pulsating with an electrifying rhythm that may leave you feeling pleasantly irregular.

Experience the exhilaration of rapid breaths.

Experience the sensation of strength slipping away as

your muscle tissues lose their power.

Introducing our revolutionary solution for excessive sweating: Say goodbye to embarrassing perspiration with our highly effective product.

Experience the sensation of a gentle tingle in your stomach, or the feeling of lightness in your bowels.

Introducing a revolutionary solution that will make it effortless to concentrate on anything else.

Introducing the all-new sensation: dizziness. Experience a whirlwind of emotions as you embark on a journey of disorientation. Brace yourself for a world that spins and twirls, leaving you breathless and captivated. Get ready to embrace the dizziness and let it take

Experience the sensation of being completely immobilized in the most captivating way imaginable. Feel the icy grip of stillness as it takes hold of your very being. Prepare to be mesmerized by the overwhelming sense of being frozen to the location.

Introducing a delectable delight that's not meant for

consumption.

Experience the ultimate sensation of hot and chilly sweats.

Experience the sensation of a parched mouth and the feeling of muscles pulled tight.

Experience the incredible phenomenon that unfolds within your body when fear takes hold. Your body, ever vigilant, springs into action, readying itself for any potential crisis. Witness as your blood circulation surges, delivering vital nutrients to your muscles, empowering them for action. Feel the surge of energy as your blood sugar levels rise, fueling your every move. And marvel at the heightened mental acuity that allows you to focus solely on the perceived threat at hand. Your body, a masterful guardian, ensures you are prepared for whatever challenges may come your way.

Experience the transformative power of overcoming anxiety. In the journey ahead, you may encounter some of the symptoms mentioned above, accompanied by a persistent sense of Fear. Prepare to conquer sleepless nights, persistent headaches, and difficulties in focusing on work and planning for the future. Rest assured, your intimate relationships may be affected, and your self-confidence may waver. But fear not, for there is hope for a brighter tomorrow.

Experience the inexplicable sensation of feeling on edge without any actual threat. Discover the intriguing reasons behind your personal unease, even in the absence of real danger.

Experience the power of swift and unwavering responses that fear ignites. In the early days, our ancestors relied on these instinctive reactions to navigate treacherous situations. But times have changed, and the threats we encounter in our modern lives are vastly different.

Discover the fascinating truth that lies within us all. It's no surprise that our thoughts and bodies continue to function just as our early ancestors did. Experience the undeniable connection as we navigate the modern world, facing the same reactions to everyday concerns such as bills, travel, and interpersonal situations. Uncover the timeless essence that unites us across generations. But wait, why should we try to escape from or assault these problems? Let's face them head-on and find the solutions we need!

Experience the overwhelming power of fear, as it grips your very being. The mysterious origins of these intense sensations only add to the terror, leaving you questioning their validity. Are they truly warranted, or do they simply exaggerate the situation at hand? Introducing a revolutionary approach: Instead of merely notifying you of potential dangers, imagine a world where your Fear or panic becomes a powerful force, capable of triggering responses to even the most insignificant or illusory threats.

Discover the secret to banishing your fears and reclaiming your sense of normalcy. Uncover the reasons behind why your fear persists and learn how to make it vanish completely. Say goodbye to the burden of fear and embrace a life of confidence and tranquility.

Experience the exhilarating rush of fear as you encounter

the unknown. Embrace the thrill of the unfamiliar, knowing that fear is merely a fleeting sensation.

Discover the hidden challenges that may be lurking in your day-to-day life, silently causing long-lasting problems that leave you puzzled. Uncover the mysterious source of your troubles, even if you can't quite pinpoint why they persist. Experience the relentless grip of anxiety, an ever-present force that haunts the lives of many individuals, without warning or reason.

Experience the multitude of fear-inducing triggers that permeate everyday life. Unravel the enigmatic nature of your fears, as their origins remain elusive. Gauge the uncertain probability of potential harm lurking in the shadows. Discover the fascinating power of the human brain as it continues to send danger signals to the body, even when fears may seem out of proportion. Witness the incredible psychological mechanisms at play, constantly alerting us to potential threats.

Discover the powerful methods to conquer Fear, both mentally and physically.

Discover the truth behind Panic Attack.

Experience the overwhelming power of an anxiety attack as it engulfs your mind and body with a torrent of fear and stress. Discover the telltale signs of this intense emotional rollercoaster by exploring the comprehensive list provided under 'What do anxiety and stress feel like?' Experience the overwhelming sensation of anxiety? Many individuals describe it as a struggle to catch their breath, accompanied by a deep-seated fear of having a heart attack or losing control of their own body. Discover the invaluable 'Support and Information' section nestled at the conclusion of this booklet, offering a lifeline for those seeking assistance in managing anxiety attacks.

Discover the fascinating world of Phobia

Discover the fascinating world of phobias, where an ordinary fear transforms into an extraordinary obsession. Experience the gripping intensity of an individual's extreme concern, whether it be towards a particular animal, thing, place, or situation. Brace yourself for a journey into the depths of the human psyche, where fears take on a life of their own. Discover the fascinating world of phobias, where individuals are driven by an insatiable desire to escape fear, sever any ties to the root cause of their stress and anxiety, and evade the clutches of fear itself. Experience the overwhelming sensation of anxiety and panic at the mere thought of encountering the source of your phobia.

Discover the Telltale Signs of When You Require Assistance

Experience the occasional bout of anxiety and stress? You're not alone. These common challenges can impact us all from time to time. Discover the true nature of mental conditions when they reach a severe and long-lasting state, as defined by medical professionals. Are you constantly feeling overwhelmed and stressed? Do your worries seem to consume your every waking moment? If so, it may be time to seek assistance from a trusted healthcare professional. Don't let stress control your life any longer - take the first step towards a happier, more balanced existence by reaching out to your physician today. Discover the power of overcoming phobias and anxiety attacks that are holding you back from living your best life.

Discover the Power of Self-Help!

Embrace the Power of Confronting Your Fears

Don't let fear hold you back from pursuing your desires and responsibilities. By constantly evading intimidating situations, you risk missing out on valuable experiences. Discover the untapped potential of facing your fears head-on. By avoiding the opportunity to test the worst-case scenario, you miss out on the chance to conquer your worries and diminish your anxiety. Don't let fear hold you back - embrace the challenge and unlock your true potential. Experience the undeniable rise of anxiety when you step into this captivating set-up. Discover the transformative power of embracing your fears and anxieties as a means to conquer stress.

Discover the power within you

Discover the fascinating depths of your fear or panic. Experience the power of self-awareness by keeping an exquisite anxiousness diary or thought record. Capture the moments when anxiety strikes and delve into the intricate details of your thoughts and emotions. Discover the power of self-assessment and unlock your potential to make a positive impact on the environment. By setting realistic goals and confronting your fears head-on, you can achieve remarkable results. Take control of your journey towards a greener future today! Introducing the ultimate solution for those prone to fear and stress: a handy summary of essential items to bring along. Never be caught off guard again! Discover the transformative power of this remarkably effective method for addressing the deep-rooted values that lie at the heart of your stress and anxiety. Discover the intriguing depths of your Fear or nervousness. Experience the power of preserving every moment and capturing every detail with our cutting-edge archiving solution. Never miss a beat as you effortlessly document when it happens and what unfolds before your eyes. Embrace the art of keeping memories alive with our innovative archival technology.

Get ready to transform your body and elevate your fitness

game with the power of exercise. Discover the incredible benefits of incorporating regular physical

Elevate your productivity with an increased number of tasks to conquer. Experience the transformative power of this engaging activity, as it captivates your attention and effortlessly lifts the weight of anxiety and stress from your mind.

Experience ultimate relaxation

Discover the transformative power of relaxation techniques to conquer the overwhelming grip of fear, both in your mind and body. Experience the incredible benefits of simply dropping your shoulder blades and taking a deep breath. Transport yourself to a serene oasis with your imagination. Discover the transformative power of activities like yoga, meditation, and therapeutic massage. Immerse yourself in the soothing wisdom of the Mental Health Foundation's wellbeing podcasts. Elevate your well-being and unlock your true potential.

Discover the Power of Healthy Eating

Indulge in a bountiful array of luscious fruits and vibrant vegetables, while steering clear of the perils of excessive sugar consumption. Experience the power of stabilizing your blood sugar levels and say goodbye to anxious feelings. Discover the secret to a stress-free life by avoiding excessive consumption of tea and espresso. Unleash your inner tranquility by steering clear of the stimulating effects of caffeine. Discover the secret to a healthier lifestyle: steer clear of excessive alcohol consumption, or indulge in moderation.

Experience the common practice of reaching for a drink when those nerves start to kick in. Discover the fascinating world of alcoholic beverages, often referred to as 'Dutch courage'. But beware, as the aftermath of indulging in these libations can leave you feeling more fearful and anxious than ever before.

Discover the Power of Complementary Therapies

Discover the power of complementary therapies and exercises to conquer anxiety. Unleash the potential of rest techniques, meditation, yoga, or t'ai chi to help you effectively cope with the challenges of anxiety.

Discover the power of faith and spirituality.

Discover a profound sense of connection to something greater than yourself through the power of faith. Discover the power of trust in navigating the challenges of daily life. Immerse yourself in the uplifting atmosphere of chapels and other trust organizations, where you can forge invaluable connections with a supportive network.

Discover the Ultimate Solution to Getting the Help You Need!

Discover the Power of Talking Therapies

Discover the incredible power of talking therapies, such as counseling or Cognitive Behavioural Therapy, in helping individuals overcome panic problems. One innovative approach is Computerized Cognitive Behavioural Therapy, which guides you through a series of self-help exercises right on your screen. Experience the transformative benefits today. Unlock a world of possibilities by visiting our GP today. Explore the endless opportunities that await you. Don't miss out on the chance to discover more. Schedule your appointment now.

Discover the power of medication.

Experience the power of drug treatments that provide immediate relief, focusing on alleviating symptoms rather than merely scratching the surface of anxiety disorders. Discover the unparalleled power of drugs when they are expertly combined with other cutting-edge treatments and unwavering support. Experience the transformative potential that lies within this dynamic synergy.

Acknowledgements

Behold the magnificent triumph of this extraordinary book, a testament to the divine intervention of God Almighty and the unwavering love and support of my cherished Family, devoted Fans, avid Readers, loyal Customers, and dear Friends. Their ceaseless encouragement has paved the way for this resounding success.